My Daily Sparkle
...of Gratitude

A Journal to Brighten Your Day

by Dr. Christine Sauer

Find more about Dr. Christine Sauer and all her contact information on the last 2 pages of this book.
For **Bonus resources,** go to:
https://SparkleSisters.org/bonuses
Email: info@DocChristine.com

Copyright © 2022 DocChristine Coaching Inc.
Book 1 of the Series: My Daily Sparkle
All rights reserved

No part of this book may be reproduced, or stored in a retrieval system, or transmitted in any form or by any means, electronic, mechanical, photocopying, recording, or otherwise, without express written permission of the publisher.

e-Book ISBN: 978-1-7773788-4-4
Paperback ISBN: 978-1-7773788-3-7

Cover design by: 100Covers

BONUSES

www.SparkleSisters.org/bonuses

Extra support for women who want to overcome their challenges, improve their mental and physical health, let go of past hurts, enjoy the present and live forward:

- Free support call with the Author
- Free LifeTime Membership in the #SparkleSisters Community

To redeem, go to: https://SparkleSisters.org/bonuses

About this book:

A keen appreciation for yourself and the world around us and a deep feeling of gratitude are some of the most important attitudes and skills every woman interested in personal growth needs to develop and grow, and a science-backed key to true and lasting happiness.

This journal is the first of a series of journals designed to help women re-gain the sparkle in their eyes and the spring in their steps.

You will find not only instructions on how to journal in a way that supports your mental well-being, but also get access to bonus resources to support your further personal growth.

About the Author:

Dr. Christine Sauer – Christine - is a German-trained physician and naturopath, a Brain and Mental Health Professional and Coach- and a Mental Health "Thriver" herself.

After nearly losing her own life through suicide, she decided that a life of sadness, fear and despair was not the life she wanted for herself and others.

She then dedicated her life to helping other women struggling with life to overcome their challenges, grow as a person, and live with energy, passion and purpose and to truly Recover Your Sparkle.

As founder of the community of ambitious women who want a sparkle in their eye and a spring in their step, to grow as people, to give and receive support, understanding and practical tools, she has truly become a #SparkleSister.

Learn more and join the community:
www.SparkleSisters.org

What is Gratitude?

Gratitude is an emotion that comes from appreciation. It's an awareness, a thankfulness of the good things in your life, in you and in the world around you.

Gratitude is a powerful thing. It can turn any negative into a positive.

It can change how you feel inside.
It can bring hope and happiness.
It can improve your health, your relationships, your career and so much more. It can literally transform your life.
So often in today's society, the negative is sensationalized and the positive is ignored. You see it in the news, in magazines and newspapers. You hear it in the grocery store, at work and even from family and friends. All of this negativity can be overwhelming to the point of wearing a person down.

If you're feeding into the negativity, if you're focusing on the negative rather than the positive, you are doing yourself a serious disservice.

You are harming your emotional wellbeing as well as your physical body.

You could be straining your relationships, hurting your career and much more.

Benefits of Gratitude

When you express gratitude, it diminishes negativity in a powerful way.

Scientific studies show that practicing gratitude leads to:

A feeling of optimism, joy and satisfaction.
Less stress, anxiety and depression.
A strengthened immune system.
Lower blood pressure.
The ability to bounce back quicker after a traumatic event.
Stronger relationships.
A feeling of being connected to your community.
Feeling less victimized by others or by life.
Being able to recognize and appreciate what you have rather than what you don't.
You becoming more compassionate and empathetic.
A better quality and more rewarding life.

Practicing gratitude changes your perspective on life.

How to Practice Gratitude

One of the easiest, and most effective ways to learn to appreciate things and practice gratitude is to keep a journal of all the things you appreciate and are grateful for every day.

You may be surprised how many items you can find when you just look for them.

Whether you choose to journal in the morning, or at night, or both is up to you.

Pick a quiet time and spend a few minutes thinking about, documenting and appreciating the positive things in your life, the positive things about the people in your life and more.

marriages have been transformed by just one partner doing this.

(Idea: Share your journal after 1 year with your loved one and give it as an anniversary or birthday gift)

Do it for a month, two months, six months or more.

The longer you do it, the more ingrained it will become in your mind and the more your thoughts will shift.

At first, recognizing the positive aspects may feel awkward, but the more you look for it, the more you will find.

There is beauty all around you. There is beauty within you.
A smile, a sunset, a friend, a personal goal being met.
These are all things you can be grateful for.
Even if you only find one thing to be grateful for each day, that's okay.
There is no right or wrong when it comes to journaling.

As you journal, try to work up to three, five or even ten things a day when possible.

The following book gives you 90 pages of journaling space to write on.
Every page has a prompt, a quote or a question for you to ponder when it comes to gratitude. Feel free to add your own ideas and thoughts. This is YOUR Journal!

Don't try to be perfect or get it right. There is no right or wrong way to practice gratitude.

The practice itself is where the power resides.

Any questions?
Contact me at info@DocChristine.com
www.SparkleSisters.org

I am grateful for you - Christine

Let's Get Started!

The next Pages will each have a quote or a question to help you get started to write in your journal.

Below it is space for your ideas.

Feel free to doodle, add your own thoughts and ideas and more.

Jump around the pages, and write down the thoughts that come to your mind as you read a question, a quote or a thought.

I always recommend adding the date, so you can later review your entries and celebrate your progress!

You are AWESOME!

Think about a recent hardship. What positive aspect or opportunity came from it?

List five things you love about yourself and why.

Write about a time when you really felt appreciative of something or someone in your life

Write about your favorite season

Think back to the past year or two. Write about some of the changes you've made and why you are grateful for them.

Write about something you love doing and why you are grateful to be able to do it.

List five positive aspects of your community and why you love them.

Sunrise or Sunset? Which is your favorite and why?

Write about how you felt the last time someone did a kind deed for you.

Write about something that makes you belly laugh.

> "Saying thank you is more than good manners. It is good spirituality."
> ~ Alfred Painter

"Gratitude turns what we have into enough.

> *"God gave you a gift of 86,400 seconds today. Have you used one to say "thank you?"*
> *~ William A. Ward*

"Silent gratitude isn't much use to anyone." ~ Gertrude Stein

"If the only prayer you said in your whole life was, "thank you," that would suffice." ~ Meister Eckhart

"If you count all your assets, you always show a profit." ~ Robert Quillen

> "There are two kinds of gratitude – The sudden kind when we receive and the deeper kind when we give."

"The struggle ends when the gratitude begins." ~ Neale Donald Walsch

> "Replace fear with gratitude, and the whole world changes." ~ Terri Guillemets

> "Hem your blessings with thankfulness so they don't unravel."

"Gratitude is the memory of the heart." ~
Jean Baptiste Massieu

"Some people grumble that roses have thorns. I am grateful that thorns have roses."
~ Alphonse Karr

> *"Gratitude is the memory of the heart."* ~
> *Jean Baptiste Massieu*

> "As we express our gratitude, we must never forget that the highest appreciation is not to utter words, but to live by them." ~ *John F. Kennedy*

> "We make a living by what we get, but we make a life by what we give."
> ~ Winston Churchill

> "It is impossible to feel grateful and depressed in the same moment."
> ~ Naomi Williams

> "Kindness is a language, which the deaf can hear and the blind can see."
> ~ Mark Twain

> "Be thankful for what you have, you'll end up having more."
> ~ Oprah Winfrey

> "If we magnify blessings as much as we magnify disappointments, we would all be much happier." ~ John Wooden

When we focus on our gratitude, the tide of disappointment goes out and the tide of love rushes in." Kristin Armstrong

> "Gratitude is the most exquisite form of courtesy." Jacques Maritain

"When I wake up in the morning, I like to express my gratitude for being on the planet. That gratefulness makes me very present." *Trudie Styler*

> "We can only be said to be alive in those moments when our hearts are conscious of our treasures." Thornton Wilder

> "When I started counting my blessings, my whole life turned around." Willie Nelson

"The deepest craving of human nature is the need to be appreciated." William James

"We often take for granted the very things that most deserve our gratitude." Cynthia Ozick

"Sometimes we should express our gratitude for the small and simple things like the scent of the rain, the taste of your favorite food, or the sound of a loved one's voice." Joseph B. Wirthlin

"We learned about gratitude and humility - that so many people had a hand in our success, from the teachers who inspired us to the janitors who kept our school clean... and we were taught to value everyone's contribution and treat everyone with respect."
Michelle Obama

> "At times, our own light goes out and is rekindled by a spark from another person. Each of us has cause to think with deep gratitude of those who have lighted the flame within us."
> Albert Schweitzer

"No one who achieves success does so without acknowledging the help of others. The wise and confident acknowledge this help with gratitude." Alfred North Whitehead

> "Silent gratitude isn't very much to anyone."
> Gertrude Stein

> *"Thanksgiving is a time of togetherness and gratitude."* Nigel Hamilton

"Gratitude is when memory is stored in the heart and not in the mind." Lionel Hampton

> "I regard gratitude as an asset and its absence a major interpersonal flaw."
> Marshall Goldsmith

What are people in your life who you are grateful for?

....
....
....
....
....
....
....
....
....
....
....
....
....
....
....
....
....
....
....
....
....
....
....
....
....
....
....
....
....
....
....

> "Gratitude is one of the least articulate of the emotions, especially when it is deep." Felix Frankfurter

"Often people ask how I manage to be happy despite having no arms and no legs. The quick answer is that I have a choice. I can be angry about not having limbs, or I can be thankful that I have a purpose. I chose gratitude." *Nick Vujicic*

"Gratitude unlocks the fullness of life. It turns what we have into enough, and more. It turns denial into acceptance, chaos to order, confusion to clarity. It can turn a meal into a feast, a house into a home, a stranger into a friend. Gratitude makes sense of our past, brings peace for today and creates a vision for tomorrow." *Melody Beattie*

> "Gratitude is the fairest blossom which springs from the soul." — Henry Ward Beecher

> "When it comes to life the critical thing is whether you take things for granted or take them with gratitude." Gilbert K. Chesterton

> "Let us swell with gratitude and allow it to overwhelm us. It isn't as cliche as we make it; life truly is short. Let's spend it all lavishly wallowing in gratitude." Grace Gealey

> "Gratitude, warm, sincere, intense, when it takes possession of the bosom, fills the soul to overflowing and scarce leaves room for any other sentiment or thought." — John Quincy Adams

> "Joy is the simplest form of gratitude." Karl Barthams

What movies or TV shows are you grateful for and why?

> *"Happiness cannot be traveled to, owned, earned, worn or consumed. Happiness is the spiritual experience of living every minute with love, grace, and gratitude."* — Denis Waitley

"I don't have to chase extraordinary moments to find happiness - it's right in front of me if I'm paying attention and practicing gratitude." Brene Brown

"The root of joy is gratefulness." David Steindl-Rastley

What food did you appreciate today?

> "Let us rise up and be thankful, for if we didn't learn a lot today, at least we learned a little, and if we didn't learn a little, at least we didn't get sick, and if we got sick, at least we didn't die; so, let us all be thankful." Buddha

"If you concentrate on finding whatever is good in every situation, you will discover that your life will suddenly be filled with gratitude, a feeling that nurtures the soul." *Rabbi Harold Kushner*

"The discipline of gratitude is the explicit effort to acknowledge that all I am and have is given to me as a gift of love, a gift to be celebrated with joy." Henri Nouwenwe

"When I pray, I always thank Mother Nature for all the beauty in the world. It's about having an attitude of gratitude." *Miranda Kerr*

> "The roots of all goodness lie in the soil of appreciation." The Dalai Lama

> "It is through gratitude for the present moment that the spiritual dimension of life opens up." Eckhart Tolle

> "I acknowledge my feeling and gratitude for life by praising the world and whoever made all these things." Mary Oliver

> *"I believe in prayer. I believe in gratitude and serving people."* — Kiran Bedi

"We should honor Mother Earth with gratitude; otherwise our spirituality may become hypocritical." Radhanath Swami

"We have to fill our hearts with gratitude. Gratitude makes everything that we have more than enough." Susan L. Taylor

> "The more grateful I am, the more beauty I see." Mary Davis

What comforts of daily life are you grateful today?

"It's wonderful to be grateful. To have that gratitude well out from deep within you and pour out in waves. Once you truly experience this, you will never want to give it up." Srikumar Rao

"A smart manager will establish a culture of gratitude. Expand the appreciative attitude to suppliers, vendors, delivery people, and of course, customers." Harvey Mackay

"A person however learned and qualified in his life's work in whom gratitude is absent, is devoid of that beauty of character which makes personality fragrant." *Hazrat Inayat Khan*

> "I'm just so very lucky to be able to do what I do for a living, and giving back is a way for me to express my gratitude. I'm so lucky to be in a position to help people, and that's appealing to me."
> PewDiePieKhan

"Charity never humiliated him who profited from it, nor ever bound him by the chains of gratitude, since it was not to him but to God that the gift was made." Antoine de Saint-Exupery

"There are slavish souls who carry their appreciation for favors done them so far that they strangle themselves with the rope of gratitude." Friedrich Nietzsche

> "In most of mankind gratitude is merely a secret hope of further favors." François de La Rochefoucauld

What flavors of food are you grateful for?

"Gratitude is one of the greatest gifts we can give. And it's not a gift we often give to children. We expect it of them, but we don't necessarily give it back." *Jason Reynolds*

"Have gratitude for the things you're discarding. By giving gratitude, you're giving closure to the relationship with that object, and by doing so, it becomes a lot easier to let go." Marie Kondo

> "Gratitude is a burden, and every burden is made to be shaken off." Denis Diderot

"I'm big on manners. I'm big on politeness. I'm big on gratitude." Kate Hudson

> "I am filled with so much sincerity and gratitude to know where I came from and what I'm doing now." Antonio Brown

> "Piglet noticed that even though he had a Very Small Heart, it could hold a rather large amount of Gratitude." — A.A. Milne, Winnie-the-Pooh

> "When you know in your bones that your body is a sacred gift, you move in the world with an effortless grace. Gratitude and humility rise up spontaneously." Debbie Ford

Remember the feeling of water on your skin or your body. What are you grateful about this?

What are things you feel grateful about when it comes to your body?

What outer circumstances are you grateful about today?

What are some things that initially hurt, but you are now grateful for?

What are things you learned that you are grateful for?

What could be different perspectives to be grateful for?

What pets are you grateful for?

Notice the beauty around you. What are you particularly grateful for?

What are thoughts you appreciate?

About the Author

Christine - Dr. Christine Sauer - is a German-trained physician and naturopath, a Brain and Mental Health Professional - and a Mental Health "Thriver" herself.
After nearly losing her own life through suicide, she decided that a life of sadness, fear and despair was not the life she wanted for herself and others.
She then dedicated her life to helping other women struggling with life to overcome their challenges, grow as a person, and live with energy, passion and purpose and to truly Sparkle.
As founder of the community of ambitious women who want a sparkle in their eye and a spring in their step, to grow as people, to give and receive support, understanding and practical tools, she has truly become a #SparkleSister

Dr. Christine Sauer also has further education in integrative and funcitonal nutrition, gastrointestinal health, orthomolecular medicine (supplements), integrative treatment of depression and other mental health issues, in neuroscience, coaching science and arts and more...

Major Certifications:
German-trained physician (dermatologist, allergologist)
German-trained naturopath
Certified Brain and Mental Health Professional (Dr. Daniel Amen MD) and Licensed Brain Trainer
Certified Havening Techniques® Practitioner (Drs. Ron Ruden MD and Steven Ruden DDS)
Licensed Neuroencoding Specialist (Dr. Joseph McClendon III).
She is part of the Teaching Teams of Dr. Amen and Dr. McClendon.

As "The Doctor Who KNOWS How You Feel" her clients value the deep personal connection she forms with them as well the practical strategies, vast knowledge and her sense of humor.

She is the founder of DocChristine Coaching and The #SparkleSisters as well as the
"The Brain and Success System" – Strategies for a Better Brain, a Happier Life and a Better Business.
Author of:
"Eating for Vibrant Health and Explosive Energy"
"The F-Word Diet"
Co-Author of:
"Raising the Bar"
"BLU Talks Vol. 04" (Business, Life, Universe)
"Invisible No More – Invincible Forevermore" (International #1 Bestselling Book)

As an engaging, inspirational and entertaining speaker, Dr. Christine has appeared on many stages, video shows and her own webinars and videos.
Her Podcast and Video Show: "Your Quality of Life - Healthy Alternatives" features conversations with fascinating people from all walks of life.

DocChristine is also active on Facebook, YouTube and LinkedIn.

Websites:
https://DocChristine.com (Main Personal Website)
https://SparkleSisters.org
https://BrainandSuccess.com
contact: info@docchristine.com